Why We Get Fat Today

Taking Positive Actions Toward Elimination

By Cathy Wilson
Copyright © 2013

Income Disclaimer

This book contains business strategies, marketing methods and other business advice that, regardless of my own results and experience, may not produce the same results (or any results) for you. I make absolutely no guarantee, expressed or implied, that by following the advice below you will make any money or improve current profits, as there are several factors and variables that come into play regarding any given business.

Primarily, results will depend on the nature of the product or business model, the conditions of the marketplace, the experience of the individual, and situations and elements that are beyond your control.

As with any business endeavor, you assume all risk related to investment and money based on your own discretion and at your own potential expense.

Liability Disclaimer

By reading this book, you assume all risks associated with using the advice given below, with a full understanding that you, solely, are responsible for anything that may occur as a result of putting this information into action in any way, and regardless of your interpretation of the advice.

You further agree that our company cannot be held responsible in any way for the success or failure of your business as a result of the information presented in this book. It is your responsibility to conduct your own due diligence regarding the safe and successful operation of your business if you intend to apply any of our information in any way to your business operations.

Terms of Use

You are given a non-transferable, "personal use" license to this book. You cannot distribute it or share it with other individuals.

Also, there are no resale rights or private label rights granted when purchasing this book. In other words, it's for your own personal use only.

Table of Contents

Why We Get Fat Today

Taking Positive Actions Toward Elimination

By Cathy Wilson

Introduction

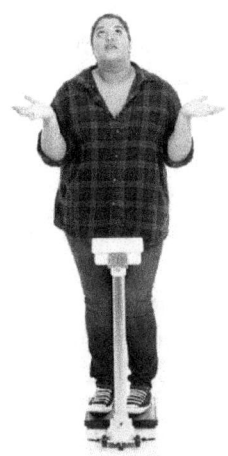

Fat is something that seems to be universally negative. Fat leads to imbalances physically, mentally, socially - it affects all aspects of life. Fat is incredibly powerful and has the ability to toy directly with emotion, the length of time you will stay on earth, and the quality of life in which you will lead.
Fat is all powerful.

Fat can steal your energy and take away your self- esteem. It can flip your attitude from positive to negative in one tub of ice cream, and twist and turn your hormones to leave you crying one minute and overjoyed the next.

Fat is an interference.
Fat will stand in the way of your happiness. Achieve your goals, enjoying life, challenging yourself for the better and living a long, healthy and prosperous life. Fat robs people of life fulfillment.

It only makes sense we should all look to understand what exactly fat is, why we need, why most of us could stand to lose a few pounds, and look to gain a positive perspective on how we can go about doing this.

You can gather every single iota of information on fat available, but if you don't have the knowledge of "how to" take action, and the drive to apply it, then what's the use? Wow, talk about a wasted encyclopedia of useless information!

My goal is to introduce fat to you in the basics, help you understand the role it plays in your life, and show you how you can take control of your fat so you can gain better overall health. You deserve to be happy and having the ability to control your fat is definitely a step in the right direction.

If you can learn one piece of useful information from this book that's going to help you make positive health changes in your life, then I've done my job.
Are you ready to get started?

What Is Fat and Why We Need It - The Science Behind It

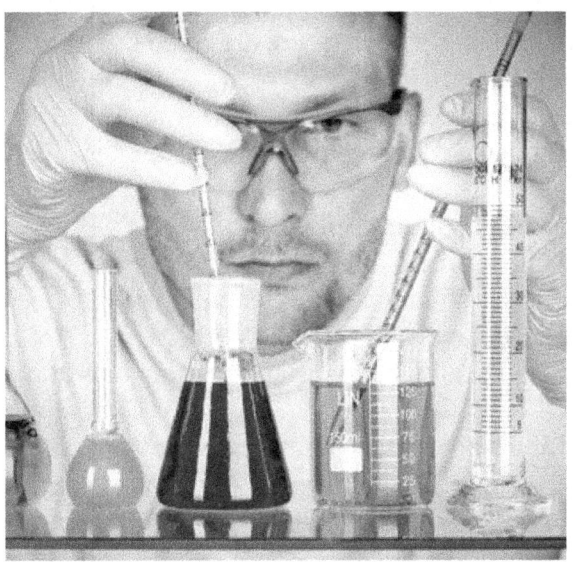

Fat Explained

Do you really know what fat is? When I think of fat I picture wiggly-jiggly cottage cheese legs or arms, rolls that tend to gather around the midsection. These are always attached to negative feelings, eternal sluggishness that may or may not mentally or physically trigger turmoil, perhaps even death eventually. Fat is linked to pretty much every single serious disease or illness out there. Which makes it even sadder because this means all of it is preventable. Diabetes, heart disease, and stroke are just a few of these qualified diseases, devestatingly true.

Fat Facts:

* Fat is a nutrient. Something you need to survive. Your body needs fat to run optimally. If your body didn't get/have fat you

wouldn't be alive. It supplies your body with energy and encourages other vital nutrients to fulfill their function which determines your health and wellness.

* Fats are a wide group of compounds that normally break down in organic compounds but not in water, soluble and insoluble respectively.

* Taking the chemical angle. Fats are recognized as tri-esters of fatty acids and glycerol. There are three different chemical ester groups.

* Fats can be found in liquid or solid forms. Olive oil and butter are examples. Room temperature fats are usually called oils and fats if they are solid.

* Lipids are fats liquid or solid.

* Fats are either oils, fats, or lipids.

     -Oils are any fat at room temperature that don't mix with water and have a greasy feel.

     - Fats are all fats but usually various fats at room temperature.

     - Lipids are universal fats, liquid or solid in state.

* Main types of fat are animal and vegetable.

     -Examples of animal fats are cream, butter, meat fat and lard

     -Examples of vegetable fats are peanut, flax, corn and olive oil.

Since when is life simple? Of course there can't be just one type of fat, in fact there are four and it's important you understand the basics of each before you venture further. To get you a little ahead in the game it's the saturated and Trans fats you want to avoid for the most part.

Saturated Fat - Technically this means each molecule of fat has hydrogen atoms. Experts agree saturated fats are linked with an increase in serious disease if this is your flavor. Too much saturated fat over a long period of time is going to increase your cholesterol number, the "bad" one, and increase your susceptibility to stroke and heart disease.

For the most part saturated fat is in animal products, including chicken skin and dairy foods. Cakes, processed foods, sweets and pastries also contain saturated fats.

Note: Coconut oil is considered a saturated fat although there are loads of positive health traits linked to it, including strengthening the immune system, clearing up skin conditions and providing energy.

So if you are having a greasy fast food meal and decide to order a rich thick shake with that and stop for a baked muffin on the way home, you are definitely overloading on the saturated fats.

Monounsaturated Fat - This type of fat is not loaded with hydrogen atoms structurally. It has room to breathe with only room for one hydrogen atom on each fat molecule. Studies show this fat is a neutral one for the most part. Meaning the impact on your health is never consistently positive or negative. The scientific based belief is that monounsaturated fats will reduce your risk for cardiovascular disease. If you've heart of the Mediterranean diet you will know it is loaded with monounsaturated fat, believed to do your body good!
Examples of monounsaturated fats are avocados, nut oil and yummy olives.

Polyunsaturated Fat - The structure of polyunsaturated fat included spaces around each fat molecule that isn't loaded with hydrogen atoms. Experts preach polyunsaturated fats to be good for our good health, particularly those found in fish, called Omega-3 polyunsaturated fatty acids. They protect us from serious preventable diseases including cardiovascular disease, along with lowering cholesterol. Symptom relieve by getting adequate amounts of this fatty acid are decreasing the severity of arthritis, tightness in the joints and various skin diseases.

Polyunsaturated fats are found in things like sunflower oil, grape seed oil, oily fish and safflower oil.

When you are looking to buy packaged foods, the less ingredients there are, the better. When cooking, go for minimal amounts of polyunsaturated fat to help keep your heart healthy and body running smoothly, including the metabolizing of fats.

Trans Fat - These are what I call "fake" fats. Trans fats are manufactured and don't occur naturally. What they do is help to extend the shelf life of packaged processed foods and with very little cost. This process involves adding hydrogen to liquid vegetable oils so they are stable longer. Just meaning they aren't going to break down and go bad so quickly. Just think about the loaf of bread that lasts a month on the shelf!

These fats are never saturated and have fewer hydrogen atoms if you want the science side of things.

You DO NOT need Trans fats at all in your life, not unless you are looking to get unhealthy and fat. These fats are the worst of all fats and unfortunately one of the most widely consumed because society today is driven by convenience. Packed and processed foods that are tasty, fast and efficient are incredibly addictive and often the staple foods of choice for many.

Baked goods and pastries, donuts, cookies, margarine, deep fried foods, and tasty sweet treats are often overloaded with Trans fats. Make it a habit of reading the label of any food item you buy. If you find this variety of fat you might want to think twice before wolfing it down. Natural is always better here.
NEWFLASH!!!!
Partially hydrogenated oils is the code name for dangerous Trans fats. Don't be fooled!

How much fat does your body need attain optimal health?
* Fat is necessary in brain growth and development - 2-3 year-olds need up to 35% of food intake per day
* Kids ages 4-18 require 25-35% of their food intake per day

* Adults over 19 need from 20-35% fat of total food intake per day

Keep in mind these are just guidelines and for adults it really is quite general. For the most part we will never have issues not getting enough fat, we go extreme the other way.
You can see some fat as tissue on your body. Pretty sure you know what I'm talking about here. Your skin covers fat or adipose tissue. In women you see it in the butt area, thighs, hips and breast area in particular. For men, they tend to have it visible on the abdomen and shoulders. So now you know the basics of what fat is. It's time to move forward to the function and purpose of fat.

Fat Purpose
There may be times where you get so fed up with that you'd like to just toss it out the window and never bother with it again. Maybe if you just stopped eating fat you wouldn't be fat?

Sorry to burst your bubble but that's not how it works. Your body needs fat to function properly and believe it or not your need to eat fat in order to burn it off. Sounds a little weird but it's very true.

The thought I'd like to introduce to you is that fat is NOT bad. Open your mind to seeing the positives in fat before you pass judgment. If you aren't willing to be good with the idea of altering your fat perception a touch, it's going to be pretty difficult for you use this book to zap fat, boost energy levels, lower your risk for serious disease and flip your life meter switch to positive forever.

First I need to mention the fact that "fat" as a whole has gotten the short end of the stick. So much so that marketers have had to label particular food items "fat-free" in order to get people to buy them. We're going to have a look at why your body needs fat, how they help you and how we can get them.

You need fat because it contains various essential nutrients vital to your good health. Fat benefits are:
* creates body tissue
* makes bio-chemicals like hormones
* gives us energy
* flavors food
* helps in growth and development, particularly in brain development of young children

The other two macronutrients your body needs on a regular basis are complex carbohydrates and lean protein. Fat has twice as much energy as either of these. Energy is measured in calories per gram. Fat has 9 calories per gram, protein and carbs, 4. The purpose of visual fat is to . . .
- be utilized as stored energy
- help shape your body
- help cushion and protect your skin, absorbs bumps
- insulate your body and ensure not too much heat is lost

Of course there's fat on your body that's invisible and it's found in and around your organs.
The functions of your hidden fat are:
- to help hold cells together
- helps make up the myelin sheathes, making it possible for nerve impulses to be transmitted
- a component of vitamin D, bile, hormones and various bio-chemicals
- protects your organ from external shock

My Thoughts . . .
Fat is necessary to have on your body and to eat in your diet. You might not be really interested in the science behind fat but it's critical you understand at least the surface level because knowing how fat negatively and positively affects your body is important.

The issues arise when we take either the eating or storing of fat to the extreme. Fat is very dangerous if you chow down the wrong type or eat foods that have too much fat, and your life-style doesn't battle back for you. By this I mean lots of exercising and great life choices to help burn up calories and burn off fat, reducing the risk of serious disease and energizing yourself.

Evolution and Fat

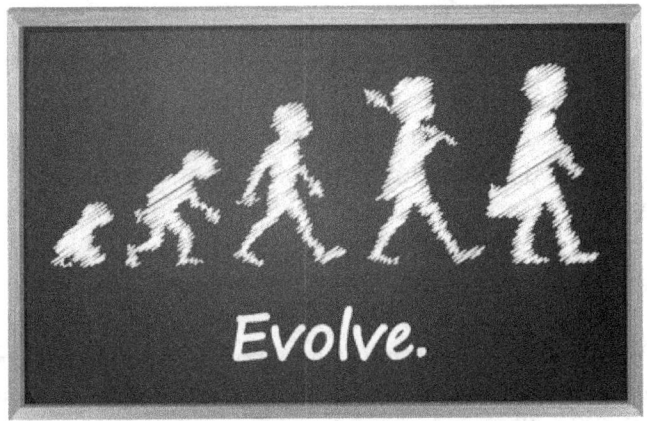

Hmmm . . . Now that's a loaded question.

Think back to the days of the "caveman.",where lives were simple, natural and pure. There were no pizza delivery boys, cell phones, cars, televisions, gaming devices and shops to make clothes and other life necessities for you.

If you look closely there are huge differences between how we live today and what "cavemen" did centuries ago with regards to:

* Nutrition
* Exercise
* Health

I'm not going deep here, seeing as this is an introductory book. But I will bring to light some of the main issues that have been triggered because we, as a society have moved so far away from days past, the way your body was programmed to function.

NUTRITION

We can look at two different aspects of nutrition here. First the fuel we are putting into our body and second the amount. Back centuries ago people didn't have very much choice in what they ate, fresh game, fruits and vegetables, herbs, wild grass, fish and numerous other all-natural foods. Nothing was processed, boxed, came in packaging or had toxic chemicals, preservatives and serious Trans fats added. The body was given the essential proteins, good carbs, vitamins and essential minerals it required to function optimally because there was nothing else. People at all natural healthy and nutrient dense foods because that's what they had, setting their body to work smoothly and without interference every day.

"Cavemen" people didn't have to worry about eating chemicals and toxins that weren't good for their body because it wasn't available. Not like we have today with all the processed foods we have at every quick market corner, grocery store and fast food joint.

Years ago people didn't have to worry so much about eating so much because they listened to their bodies. They didn't have interference like we do today; environmentally, mentally, socially, medically, and physically to start. People were in tune with what their body was saying. If their tummy was rumbling they would fill it, not register this as a sign of losing weight, like we do today.

A body that gets the right nutrients in plenty is a happy body. One that will work hard to stay healthy and strong because it "knows" the person is taking care to feed it properly, there is trust. Of course we do nothing of the sort. We stress and deprive our bodies so much each day. We skip meals, work through hunger pains, eat all the wrong foods, and basically message our body that we really don't care. We do not treat our body with respect and in return it most certainly does its best not to listen when it comes time to lose weight, get slim and toned and healthy.

Why should it?

Today we have too many "wrong" food choices at our fingertips which are extremely addictive and habitual. This is very dangerous in the game of life. Could you imagine how differently we would be living our lives if we could only eat completely all natural foods. Do you think our health in general would be better? You bet your bottom dollar it would!

If you aren't eating healthy and nutritious foods in the right amounts you are going to get fat, that's a fat fact.

EXERCISE

We are a lazy society. Electronic gadgets, cars, couches, televisions, restaurants, grocery stores, desk jobs and fast food delivery are just a few prime examples of silent "killers" in our society. The body was designed to have regular physical activity. It works best if you keep it moving, in shape and energetic, strong and resilient.

Centuries ago "the physical" was in every single thing. If people wanted to survive and stay strong they had to be physical. If you wanted to eat, sleep, keep warm and live to see another day you had to be physically strong.

When you were hungry you had to eat. This also helped to fight off disease and keep you one step ahead of becoming lunch for an enemy tribe or hunting animal. The weak did not survive. Hunger meant you needed to go out and physically exert yourself to track and capture some game. This would feed you, your family and tribe. If you didn't exercise and cleverly outwit an animal or two, then you wouldn't eat and likely wouldn't survive. This happened quite frequently back in the day.

So you used your muscles and elite cardiovascular endurance to capture and kill wild game, drag it back to camp, clean and cook it before you even got to fill your belly. A whole lot of crazy physical exercise and you would get rewarded after all this with a nice full belly. Soon after because your body was so strong and needed so much all natural food to stay this way, you would need to go right back out and do it again. In fact centuries ago people were trying to find time to rest their bodies enough.

It's the opposite today. We "rest" way too much and look to schedule a few minutes of "ho-hum" exercise a few days a week as an afterthought. Backwards don't you think?
Because of the "lazy" way in which we live today it's even more important we make the time to get intense physical into our day. As much as we can will never really be enough,, but some is better than nothing.

Let me ask you something. Do you think when an older man with a bad hip had a tiger chasing him years ago that he told the tiger not to bother chasing him for lunch because he just wasn't feeling up to running faster than he ever had in his life today? I think not! Centuries ago people just didn't make excuses, proving that a body at any age and in any condition will benefit with exercise.

We are so lazy today that we actually believe our excuses not to put physical activity into our day, even the physical activity that's a lazy activity. It's like going for a nice slow stroll for an hour, or how about riding our bike slower than a turtle and calling it exercise.

We have re-programmed our brains to be okay with not giving our body the basic physical activity it needs to survive strong, energetic and agile. We really should be ashamed of ourselves. No wonder we have so many health issues. Aches and pains, sickness and disease, most of which truly are preventable, but we don't seem to care. It's no wonder we get fat.

Without burning excess energy off your body has no choice but to store it as fat. When we are feeding our body foods that aren't natural, this makes it even easier to get fat because your body doesn't know how to get rid of it. These processed foods, toxins and preservatives interfere with your normal metabolic process and this means you are going to pack on more fat and have a tougher time getting rid of it. It doesn't take a rocket scientist to figure that one out.

It's no wonder we are getting fat!

HEALTH

Do you think people centuries ago were healthier mind and body than we are today? That's a huge YES.

Sure there weren't medicines out there to help people survive serious disease. So something like widespread smallpox could wipe out a whole tribe. But for the most part they were healthier because they didn't create health issues like we do today, then bandage them with medications and prescriptions that only manifest more issues of miscommunication within the body. Do you see where I'm going with this?

As a society we don't feed our bodies adequately and we don't keep our mind and body strong with regular strenuous and challenging physical activity. This will eventually manifest in PREVENTABLE diseases, for the most part anyway.

Centuries ago people faced different challenges than us today. Most involved a physical release and serious threat to survival. The mental was taken care of because a physical release of stress was something practiced "without though" each day.

Today, we rarely use the physical to deal with built up stress. Instead we might plop on the couch and eat a whole tub of ice cream. Sure this might make us feel better for a minute, the overwhelming short-lived spike in our blood sugar levels from nutrition-less simple carbs, but all it does is create more stored stress. These stresses take their toll on our health over time. Manifesting into disease over time and poor health.

23

If you aren't functioning optimally mentally, physically and emotionally, you are going to create stress, disease, and fat.

My Thoughts . . .
Simple really is better when it comes to good health and the people of the past have proven this exercising regularly and making sure we deal with our stresses, mainly self-created, we are not going to be healthy and part of this is being fat.
We are a fat society and the fault is all our own. Like it or lump it. You can laze your life away on your couch eating ding-dongs or you can take action, get rid of fat and build your mental physical and emotional strong. We need to steer back towards the simpler way of living if we want to lose fat and get healthy.

Why? The Emotional/Psychological of Fat

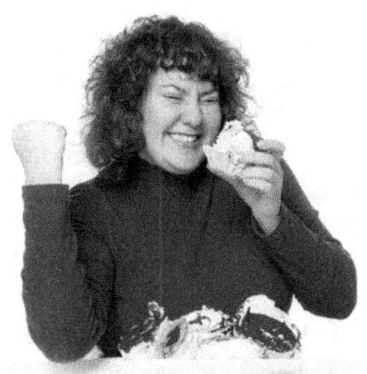

Unfortunately we seem to eat for every reason other than eating because we are hungry. We eat for emotional and psychological reasons that contribute to getting fat. Here are a few reasons people eat:
* bored
* anxious
* depressed
* sad
* stressed
* worried
* social pressures
* relationship issues
* celebration
* rebellion

There are so many emotional/psychological reasons we eat that unfortunately have become habit. We have then created an even bigger issue because we aren't even conscious of our reason for eating unneeded foods. If we have a fight with our boyfriend we head straight to the candy store to fill our face. When we are depressed because we may have gotten fired or perhaps lost a loved one, we are programmed to find comfort in lazing around and eating foods that have loads of fat and calories and very little nutritional goodness. None of which is going to keep us slim and healthy.

Here are a few factors the experts agree contribute to getting fat:
* Lazy Habits - Couch potatoes prove this one for certain: Three hundred years ago men at least 150 calories less every day and women 300. Children were out running around rather than sitting inside playing games on the computer and watching television. These habits that increase the likelihood of getting fat. Kids in general are more likely to stay indoors and eat, rather than get active and do everything but eat.

* Television and Media - Unfortunately there are loads of influential people that shape our actions on a daily basis. Take celebrities for instance. If you happen to love the infamous golfing icon Tiger Woods, and you see he wears Nike, you might also buy the product just because he does. When it comes to eating people are self and socially conditioned to do the exact same thing. These supposed "role models" can influence young people into getting addicted to high-calorie soda and unhealthy chips just because they have commercials on television with these glorified celebrities eating these "bad" foods and still looking beautiful. Gone is the realism in our brains because we want so badly to believe we can eat unhealthy but tasty foods and still look fabulous.

Packaging and consistent pressure by the advertising media out there also contribute directly to our "fat" society. They really don't give a crap about your health or the health of your family. All they really care about is making more money, even if it's at the direct expense of your financial security and good health. It's just not worth it.

* Home Environment - In our society we've come to use unhealthy sweets and pastries as "rewards" for behaving, particularly with young people. Grandma and Grandpa might spoil the kids with high fat treats when they visit and parents often turn to packaged and convenient foods to feed the children because they are so busy trying to make ends meet. Fast food restaurants are really tempting when you've worked a 60 hour week and just don't have any energy or time to feed your starving children. This is going to increase the fat-factor in your household.

* Addictions - Did you know that if you choose to snack of treats when your tummy is rumbling, that you're actually teaching yourself to crave the unhealthy when you really do need to eat? You should always go for something healthy when you are truly hungry first, fill yourself up with the vitamins and minerals your body needs, and if you're still hungry after you can have a bit of a treat. This way you will better control your unhealthy cravings and keep the balance tipped toward moderation. Food is one addiction we seem to battle as a society today, another than contributes directly to fat gain is alcohol.

* Emotional Issues Due To Work - Kids crave attention from their parents and rightly so. But because of the greediness of our world today, moms and dads are required to work crazy hours in order to deliver the "basics" in life to their children. This means a whole lot less time actually home with children. Kids end up with more confusion, less support and more emotional turmoil to deal with in general, just because. This is stressful and we all know that stress his dangerous when it comes to gaining fat and getting unhealthy. We have more emotionally unstable children in our world today because of the stresses to work on the parents, which keeps them away from their children. The connection is weaker and kids have to

make more grown-up decisions earlier in life they just aren't mature enough to make.

For instance, is a child going to grab a back of chips for dinner or try and make a pot roast with sweet potato and veggies? Need I say more?

What's important here is that we recognize what this all does to the confidence and self-esteem of both kids and adults. If we aren't able to deal with the stresses of everyday life and start to pile on the pounds, turning to embarrassing emotional eating and becoming lethargic and depressed because of it, then how can we expect to be healthy? Well we can't. It's a never-ending circle of chaos that will never change until we recognize our destructive habits and those of our children, and set out to change them.

A little further in the book we will look at answers to our fat issues of today. The peace of mind knowing there is an answer to our unwanted fat is the first step in taking action to get rid of it.

My Thoughts . . .
The emotional/psychological factors in life are hugely reflective of our excess fat and unhealthy lifestyles in general. When people get emotionally stressed they often look to food as an escape. Unfortunately we usually aren't programmed to drown our sorrows in a bag of carrots, but rather a tub of ice cream of whole chocolate cake. It's not until we start to recognize our destructive eating habits and lazy lifestyle choices, will we ever have the know-how to actually make the lifestyle health changes we need to in order to positively drop fat and get healthy for the long-term. This takes a whole lot of courage and don't worry because I'm not here to judge. Just help you recognize that if you want to get rid of your fat you can. You've just first got to face it, accept it, and work at creating a plan to make it happen - NO EXCUSES!

Fat And The Physical

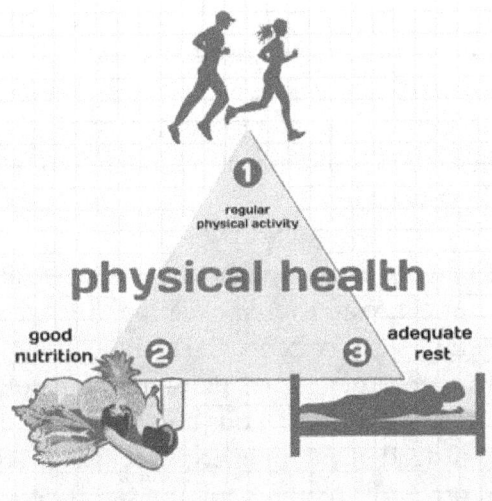

If you want to lose fat and keep it off, you've got to make healthy food choices and get physical. We've already discussed the importance of physical activity in the importance of your overall good health. Your bodily systems need physical activity to run optimally. This helps your mental, social, physical and emotional well -being. If you want to get rid of fat and keep your fat "in check," you need regular physical activity. Getting physical burns calories and burning more calories than your body needs is going to zap your fat. The numbers are the numbers.

Your body fat is the most "dense" form of energy in your body. Fat weighs less than muscle (protein) because fat doesn't have the ability to transport water. It's a pure energy source the is quickly stored by your body for future use and the more calories you feed your body each day, regardless of whether they are "healthy" or not, the more fat you will store.

In basics, a pound of body fat has about 3,500 calories. Now this is a HUGE generalization because each body is unique in nature and there are so many factors that influence the rate in which you burn calories. This just gives you a solid platform from which to start. There are about six times more calories in a pound of fat versus a pound of muscle, which naturally makes it easier to lose your muscle compared to fat, which of course you don't want to do.

How you lose fat depends on what you eat, when and how much of it your eat, your exercise regime, lifestyle, body composition, genetics, sleep patterns and so much more. For instance, if you aren't getting enough protein in your daily diet and are trying to burn off fat. Your body is going to break down muscle instead of fat for energy because it's more readily available and protein is required to burn fat. If you aren't eating it the default in your body will look to breaking down your muscle to get the protein it needs to burn off fat. This isn't going to help you because you need to build muscle in order to burn more fat, not break it down.
A muscular body burns more calories at rest than a fat one does any day of the week.

KEYS TO BURNING FAT?

Key One - High intensity interval training while fueling your body correctly. This means intermittent cardiovascular activity with bouts of weight lifting or strength training to trigger your body to burn more fat. This means your body is going to be burning fat effectively and at a fast pace because you are forcing your body to expend maximum energy at all times. There's no time here for getting bored of memorizing your gym routine. Hard working diverse physical activity including weight training and cardiovascular activity is going to get your metabolism up and this means fat is going to get zapped, assuming you're making healthy food choices too in moderation.

Key Two - Regular physical activity is so important if you are going to burn fat. This makes sense. The more you increase your metabolism the more calories and fat you're going to burn. Physical exertion is going to boost the amount of energy your body uses. Exercise more and burn more, it's that simple, theoretically anyway.

It's important that you participate in physical activities that you enjoy. Things like biking, hiking, swimming, jogging, power walking, aerobics, boot camps, skating, cross country skiing, treadmill, elliptical trainer and the cross trainer are examples of physical activities that will get your blood pumping and heart rate up, forcing your body to burn more energy than it would if you were sitting on your fanny. As mentioned in "Key |One" it's important that you implement some weights or strength training into your regular physical exercise to make your time spent exercising more effective and efficient. This means less time to get fat loss results.

Key Three - Diversity is important in anything you do to improve your overall health and wellness, particularly when looking to reduce fat. By changing up your exercise routine you are going to encourage your body to burn more fat and calories because you aren't going to get bored, you'll force your mind and body to concentrate, you'll pay better attention to from, you will use different muscles and get faster results, and you'll feel more excited about exercise because it's always different.

My Thoughts . . .
You need to get physical activity into your day if you are serious about getting rid of fat for good. Fat stores will always be associated with how your body burns calories and how many calories it burns. If you have a physically fit body that is mus-

31

cular and efficient in burning fat, then you are less likely to carry around that spare tire or two. Your mental, social, physical and emotional well-being is dependent on you making sure you get regular physical activity in your life. You are important so don't think about it, just do it!

The Social of Fat

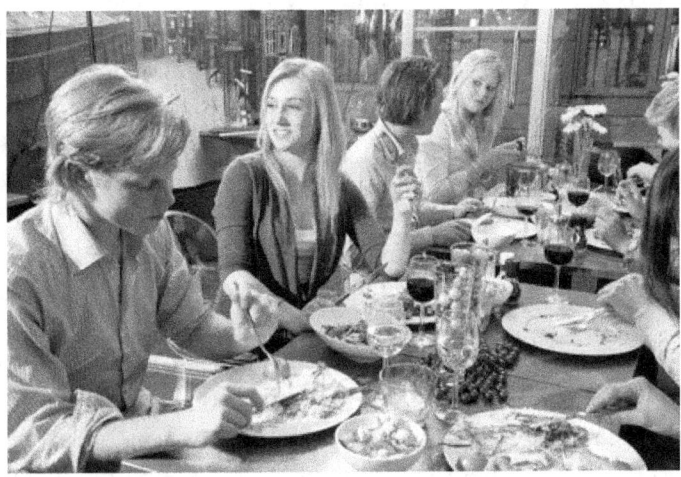

Let's face it. As humans we cave the social acceptance of others. Nobody wants to be the odd ball out and this makes it very difficult sometimes to say no, particularly when "everyone else is doing it." This is especially difficult when we are trying to make better food choices to lose weight, and the people we are being social with don't seem to care what they eat or how much.

Did you know that over one third of Americans are obese? Meaning they are more than 20% over the weight they need to be if you're going to label them healthy. It's also safe to say the majority of people that are social with overweight or obese people are likely to be the same themselves.

Humans are influential in general and studies have shown the habits of others quickly ware off or become adopted by others. So if you are the "smaller" one to start in a group of larger people, it's not surprising that you too may also get fat over time. Just think of the "monkey see, monkey do" mentality here.

This is particularly difficult when a large part of being social often involves eating and drinking. Maybe you like to go out with your friends to the movies and always order a large popcorn with double butter and a soda. Or perhaps you head out every Friday night with your friends for chicken wings and beer. Seems silly to go out and eat healthy when everyone else around you is pigging out. This is where willpower is put to the test and often challenges and makes you choose between having a good time with your friends or becoming a stick in the mud. Nobody wants to ruin the party right?

Social pressures also cause huge issues with young people because they so badly want to be accepted and loved by their peers. These fast-food lunches and junk food binges on the weekends quickie manifest into unhealthy lifelong habits that are really tough to break. We don't seem to like change as humans and when stresses occur we often fall right back into our original learned comfort zone. One of which we surround ourselves in healthy food choices and very little exercise.

Of course the social factors in life aren't the only ones that make us fat but they are definitely the ones that often challenge us the most, sending many people with great health intentions right back to the drawing board time and again. Call it sabotage or what you will, but it's something that needs to be addressed if you are looking to get rid of your extra fat and keep it off indefinitely.

My Thoughts . . .
Being social is something that all "normal" humans crave and need in order to be happy and healthy. We use the social to gain acceptance of ourselves, to find value and self-worth. To feel like we actually belong and are appreciated. Loners tend to be deviants of society with numerous acceptance issues of

themselves and society. That's a generalization and is just meant to reiterate the fact that people need people. We need social groups to exist happily and it's important that we have regular interaction with other humans on a regular basis. It's a part of our genetic makeup if we want to function optimally in our world today. This also means the social groups we interact with are going to be very influential on how we live our lives. What we eat, how much and when, along with our lifestyle preferences including exercise and wellness habits: To smoke or not to smoke: To drink or not to drink. To exercise or not and make healthy eating choices or load ourselves with junk. These are all factors that will make us fat or not.

Myths about Fat

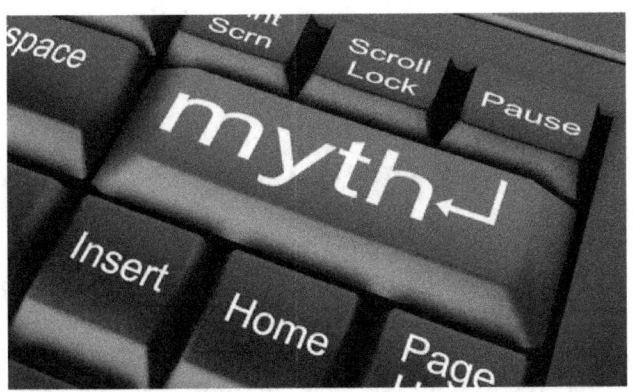

Bottom line is fat is one of the largest misunderstood foods we eat. Doesn't matter who you point the finger at here because we need to set these myths straight and make certain you have all the correct information about fat so you can make the best decisions possible when looking to get rid of yours.

Myth One - Fat is something your body just doesn't need.

Truth - Your body need fat. In fact you can't live without it. Fat is required for your nerve impulses to function properly, to insulate your organs and keep you warm, for your brain to work and to help make hormones. If you didn't have healthy fats you wouldn't have the energy you need to make it through the day, thinking would become an issue and you'd be as clumsy as heck. Healthy fats are something your body needs each day. Your survival depends on it.

Myth Two - By eating more fat you are going to get fatter.

Truth - This just isn't true. By eating more calories than your body burns you are going to gain fat.

It doesn't matter whether you are getting the extra calories from protein, carbohydrates, or fat, if you take in more energy than your body is going to use you're going to gain fat. The issue with fat is that is so dense it packs power in its punch. Meaning gram for gram fat is going to give you more calories than protein or carbs.

Myth Three - Eating low-fat is the only way you're going to zap fat.

Truth - Of course lowering the amount of fat you eat may help you burn off fat. But "low-fat" per say doesn't mean you are going to lose fat. If you chow down on an overload of low-fat foods, you can still gain fat. Keep in mind that low-fat foods are often packed with excess sugar and this can also lean towards weight gain even though they are lower in actual fat than the "real" all natural version of the same food.

These low-fat foods have also been proven to increase the odds of developing metabolic syndrome and diabetes because of the higher sugar content. Both of which don't help you lose fat. Keep moderation in mind here and make certain you find the balance of healthy food choices you need to help with your fat loss.

Myth Four - It's bad for your heart to eat saturated fats from red meats and dairy foods.

Truth - We need to be careful here because some of this myth is true. This one relies heavily on the actual health of the animal. For instance a cow that east only grass will have much leaner cuts of meat and lower fat milk than one that eats high fat grains. If a farmer is looking to fatten his cows up he will opt to fill them full of grain.
Grass fed cows also have higher CLA or conjugated linoleic acid. Studies show this is good for cancer protection and aids in weight loss. Your best bet is to be very careful the kind of meat

38

you eat and make sure when possible you opt for grass fed animals.

Myth Five - Out with the butter and in with the margarine.

Truth - The medical community as a whole is to blame for this one. The problem is that margarine contains what's referred to as Trans fats. This is a chemically created fat that is very dangerous to your health, worse than even saturated fat, which is found in butter. Trans fats are very hard on your blood vessels and build up quickly in your arteries. They also contain partially hydrogenated oils which are linked to heart disease, lowering good cholesterol and increasing bad cholesterol.

Myth Six - Cholesterol is raised by eating fat.

Truth - Cholesterol is necessary in a healthy body and many people fail to recognize they don't have a whole lot of control over their cholesterol. By eating at least three servings of fruits and veggies per day you can help protect your heart and better your cholesterol. Steering clear of bad fats is going to help with your cholesterol too. So by balancing your nutrition making all the right food choices you are going to naturally increase your good cholesterol and decrease the bad.
Tips to choose wisely here are:
- Don't overcook your vegetables because this takes away healthy nutrients
- Steer clear of fried foods
- Stay away from Trans fats
- Try to avoid partially hydrogenated oils

Myth Seven - If I was younger I could lose fat.

Truth - Yes your metabolism naturally loses some steam as you age, beginning to lower up to ten percent each year starting in your early thirties. This doesn't mean you can't lose weight if you're older though. It just means you need to pay attention to your health choices and make certain you are increasing your exercise too. Building lean muscle is key here because that can be done at any age and naturally increases the rate in which you burn calories even when you're napping.

Don't let your age determine fat loss. If you want to lose fat you can - no excuses!

My Thoughts . . .
Fat myths are something that can really much with your plans to zap fat and keep it off. Make certain you get to the bottom of anything you hear that just doesn't make sense when it comes to losing fat. If you arm yourself with the "right" information, you are going to set yourself up for fat.

Positive Action Against Fat

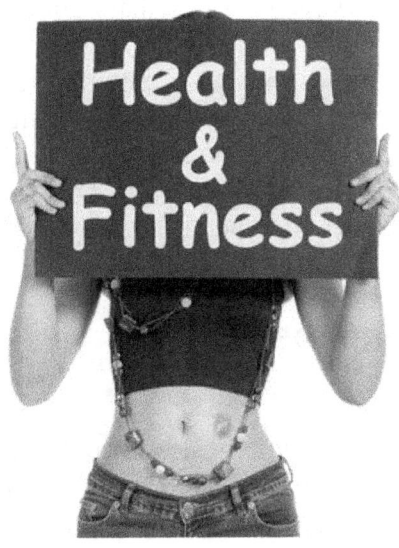

Lots of books out there are quit to point out all the negative consequences fat brings and leave you hanging with that pit of despair planted deep in your tummy and know plan of action to turn the tables.

It's important to recognize and accept you have a few extra pounds to lose but even more important to know how you are going to go about this fat loss successfully for the long run. You are NOT jumping on the "fad diet train" where you're going to fall victim to short-lived and extreme measures to lose fat. Which works for a few months before you recognize a liquid diet just doesn't work in the real world. Or that fruit really is yummy but there really are days you'd like a piece of meat or even whole grains to just change things up a touch. Fad diets set your hopes up for unrealistically fast results. We know this but want so badly to believe they work that we're will to throw our hat to the wind and try them. Again and again they fail and

41

it's time for you to wake up and take positive action to get happy with your body, mind and soul.

Set a realistic fat loss plan in place that's going to help you shed those extra rolls sensibly over time, while helping you establish new healthy habits that are going to support your hard efforts towards change. It's got to be logical and it HAS to work for you. Open your mind and expect to make a few misjudgments before you find your new normal and you will be smiling all the way to the beach if I've got anything to say about it!

HOW TO GET RID OF FAT

Commit to Change
It doesn't matter what anybody else says. If you aren't happy with your body and health, you are going t have to commit to making positive changes. It's not about going through the motions, you're better than that. You will need to first decide you want to get healthier, lose weight, make better food choices and increase your physical exercise each day.

This isn't about trying a new exercise class for a few weeks and skipping out on the sweets. This is about moderation and logic, taking small steps each and every day that work for you in order to make new healthy habits that are going to be your new healthy normal for life.

If you are serious about losing body fat and keeping it off then you will need to commit to a lifestyle change. I can definitely help you with that but only if you are going to make it happen. Anybody can be lead to water but nobody can make someone else drink it if they don't want to. If you are ready to drink then I want to help.

Open Your Mind

We are creatures of habit and we really don't think too positively of change. Even if we know our actions are not good for us we will continue to justify them until the cows come home. If you are going to be successful in losing fat you are going to have to think about lifestyle changes and look for the positive in them. You are going to have to open your thinking to making better food choices, exercising and making other positive lifestyle changes. Maybe you are a smoker and afraid that if you stop smoking you are going to gain weight?

That's fair to think but that doesn't have to happen. Remove your negative habit of smoking at your own pace and replace it with positive ones. Like finding physical exercise you enjoy, maybe picking up a new hobby or finding new friends that steer you in another direction. Where there's a will there's a way. You are important and opening your mind to making better health decisions is only going to make your life that much more enjoyable. It's all positive thinking.

Make Healthier Food Choices
Notice here I don't talk about dieting. Unfortunately before that dreaded "diet" word even rolls off the tongue you likely have thoughts of defeat and deprivation in your mind. It's a negative word associated with food stress. So let's look to establish new healthier eating habits instead. This isn't about not allowing yourself to enjoy foods that make you happy. But rather taking small steps to move towards giving your body more of the essential vitamins and minerals it requires to work more effectively and efficiently for you.

Here are a few pointers to get you started:
* Switching your white bread for whole grain - White bread is a simple carbohydrate. This means it gives you a short burst of energy because its broken down quickly, then sends your energy levels to the bottom of the barrel. Choosing a healthy whole grain bread instead if going to give your body the vitamins and minerals it requires to give you long term energy, level blood

sugars and give you the fiber you need to push toxins from your body and keep you regular. Switching to whole grain rice and pasta is also beneficial.

* Condiments can tack up loads of extra fat and calories. Condiments can turn your healthy sandwich into a high fat and high calorie meat in the snap of the fingers. Mayonnaise and other creaming dressings should be avoided if possible. It's better to put a little bit of mustard or barbecue sauce on your sandwich instead. They are nearly fat free and much lower in calories. If you must have your mayo make sure you just smear a little on instead of drowning your sandwich in it. This may seem like a very minor adjustment but it really is the small changes that add up over time.

* Salads aren't created equal. The majority of salads out there aren't healthy. Or at least we turn them into unhealthy meals. The majority of salad dressings are all fat. One tablespoon can have up to 100 calories, turning a 350 calorie healthy grilled chicken salad into a 700 calorie fat-laden meal. If you are using dress opt for fat-free. A great trick is to order the dressing on the side and just drizzle it on.

Macaroni and potato salad, or any other salad made with a creamy dressing is not good for you. If you can't help yourself just have a spoonful or two and load the rest of your plate up with wholesome fruits and vegetables for your sides.

* Stick with clear soups for a healthier choice. If you are opting for a nice hot bowl of soup make sure you aren't having a creamy type. Cream of celery, cream of broccoli, creamy tomato, and French onion soup are loaded with fat and calories that are not going to help you drop fat.
* Make sure you eat your breakfast. Studies show that people who eat breakfast are less likely to overeat later in the day. You don't drive your car on an empty gas tank and you shouldn't do this with your body either. By eating a nice light breakfast with

protein, complex carbs and essential vitamins and minerals you are giving your mind and body the energy it needs to burn fat, get energized, and keep our noggin sharp.

* It's important to get your protein. Protein is a macronutrient your body needs regularly in large amounts and doesn't manufacture or store it. This means you need to get your protein through food and having 2-3 small portions each day is your best route. Protein is a building block of life, it's in every cell, helps you build fat burning muscle and is a major contributor to your energy levels. Without adequate protein you aren't going to have very good coordination or thinking either.

* Mini meals work best for your body. You are in constant motion during the day and this means you are using energy constantly. By eating smaller healthy meals regularly you are going to help keep your blood sugar levels constant and this means less ups and downs with your moods to start. If you want your body to trust you and burn fat you need to fuel it with all the nutrients it requires and on a regular basis when it requires. This is also going to help you feel good as a whole.

Getting Physical is a HUGE Part of Blasting Fat and Keeping it off

The more physical you are on a daily basis, the more fat and calories you are going to burn. Make a conscious effort to get active during your everyday. Take the stairs instead of the elevator and park a few blocks from your destination because you can. Walk your kids to school instead of driving and how about going for a family hike on the weekends instead of sitting indoors and watching television. These are simple suggestions to get your body working harder for you and this means your fat is going to disappear sooner.

Here are a few more factors that will help you take control of your body and rid it of unwanted fat:

* Physical exercise is only going to help increase your metabolism, boost your spirits and help your body burn off excess energy stored as fat. Exercising will also help all of your internal systems run more efficiently and this means less creaks and cracks for you.

*Interval training is the fastest and most effective route to burning your fat stores. By alternating short periods of cardiovascular exercise with bouts of weights or strength training maneuvers you are going to encourage your body to burn more fat while boosting your resting metabolism. Building more muscle with the weights and increasing your respiratory is going to help you zap fat faster and burn more energy in total, even while you are sleeping.

Examples of interval training are circuit training, boot camp training and intense personal training sessions involving supersets and/or cardio activity and weight training sessions.
Note - Technique is very important in any exercising that you are doing. After getting clearance from your doctor you need to ensure you have a trainer or other fitness professional show you how to execute your training regimen correctly. This will help you to ensure you are working out effectively and that you don't hurt yourself. Sitting on the sidelines for 4-6 weeks with a strained calf muscle isn't going to help you blast fat, so please be smart about this.

* Diversity is the key when you are exercising. If you are executing the same routine at the same pace with the same exercises every single day, boredom will set in and your body isn't going to work as hard because it doesn't have to. This will cause you to lose interest and desire in exercising and you aren't going to get the results you want because your body and mind are on autopilot. By always changing things up you're going to avoid plateauing and this means effort is always going to equate to results for you, increasing the chances of you succeeding in getting healthy and zapping fat.

If you are used to biking for your cardiovascular activity try swimming or hiking. When you are doing your two x fifteen minute weight training sessions per week change up your muscles worked on a regular basis. You can also change the count, number of reps or amount of weight. These small adjustments also diversify your routine and force positive change.

There are just so many different methods of making sure you diversify your physical exercise routine. Just make sure you do this because it's only going to benefit your progress.

POINTERS TO KEEP FAT OFF

Losing fat is one thing but keeping it off for good is a whole other scenario. What's important here is that you make the positive nutrition and exercise adjustments in your life that will stand the test of time. It's not about dropping ten pounds of water weight in a week by starving your body. Only to feel defeated in adding it all back on in then some the second you eat a healthy meal. That sort of expectations is unreasonable and a surefire way to set yourself up to fail.

You need to start of smart and be willing to make minor adjustments in the foods you eat and exercising you do in your everyday, so you can set yourself up to lose fat at a steady pace without going to the extreme. Losing 1-2 pounds of fat per week with better eating and regular exercise is going to help you set yourself up to lose fat for good and feel fantastic for it. First have your mental on straight and know that you need a plan in place. One that will give you the time you need to drop fat and a program that works with h your preferences and tolerances, one that you are going to stick with for life. If you hate going to the gym then don't. Get your cardiovascular in by joining a cycling or running group. Having free weights at home and learning a strength training circuit will ensure you are building muscle while burning fat.

If you have a good knowledge of healthy eating then you are ahead of the game. Now it's time for you to start applying your knowledge. Making sure you cut down on the fats and sweets and load up on fresh fruits and vegetables, lean protein and complex carbohydrates. Drinking plenty of water along the way because dehydration will leave you feeling confused, lethargic and it will hinder your weight loss.

Here are a few pointers to help you keep fat off for the long run:

Accountability Factor
Some people are very good at taking on a new challenge and seeing it through to the end. Others needs a little bit of outside inspiration. By letting friends and family know you are going to lose fat by eating healthier and exercising more, you are increasing your chances considerably of sticking to your goals. Better yet signing up with a nutritionist and personal trainer to start is a smart move because nobody wants to throw money away and you will think twice about missing a sessions because that's just wasted money on your part.

It's a whole lot easier for most to roll over and hit the snooze button if it's just you heading to the gym to get your juices flowing. But if you are training with a partner or are part of a group session you are more likely to get your butt out of bed because if you don't there will be someone to answer to. In most cases we have no trouble disappointing ourselves but don't really want to do the same to others.

Weight Check
We need to see progress in order for our efforts to register, encouraging us to continue on with our newly learned healthy habits. By simply stepping on the scale once a week it's easy to measure progress with our weight. The flip side is we can also steer off regression backwards by recognizing early if we've slipped and need to get back on track.

Having a ceiling set weight is also a great move to keep your fat loss off. Let's say you've lost ten pounds recently and that is your "happy" weight for now. You might want to have a set weight point around there in which you don't ever want to surpass. If you do then you will immediately start playing closer attention to what you are eating, how much and when, and add a few more exercise sessions to your week.

This is just going to make certain you stay on track and don't look to regain the fat you worked so hard to take off.

Clothing Fit
This is another method in which people keep their fat loss in check, by how their clothes fit. If you happen to slip into your skinny jeans and find they are a little bit snug, this may signal for you to cut back on your sweets a little more and add an extra fifteen minutes to your cardiovascular training each week. You need to do what works for you. But clothing fit is an excellent method of ensuring you aren't becoming obsessive with your weight loss but you really are serious about it.

Diversity
Changing things up on a regular basis is going to increase your success rate with fat loss long term. In both exercising and nutrition it will starve off boredom and encourage your body to always work at maximum level in the calorie burning department. Your head will always be thinking and your muscles will always have to be ready to be challenged at a moment's notice. This just means your efforts will always equal reward and you won't ever have to worry about getting stuck in a rut.

Challenge Yourself
Going through the motions in exercising or eating isn't going to help you one bit. By challenging yourself you are going to keep inspired to stay on track to making positive lifestyle changes

that are going to result in fat disappearing, energy levels rising and diseases being deterred.

Giving your body lots of different vital nutrients is going to ensure you are getting everything you need to stay strong and healthy. While pushing yourself in your training sessions makes certain you are getting the results you want fast.

Accept You Are Human

This one is very important. You are only human and life is bound to throw a few curveballs at you. This is totally fine. You need to recognize when you veer off course and use your sheer will and determination to get yourself back on track immediately. Don't go out on a Friday night and overindulge a little, only to say you will get back to eating right and exercising Monday.

Stop yourself, accept the past as the past and get back on track now, not later. This just proves to yourself you aren't perfect but you are smart enough to recognize when you've slipped and that you are willing to do whatever it takes to get back at it. Don't focus on just the moment because it's the big picture that's really important.

My Thoughts . . .
You can have all the information you want but if you don't know how to take action with it then it really is useless. Theoretically sometimes the smartest people in the world really are the dumbest.
It's important to you take the knowledge about fat and how to lose it and apply what works for you. Understand your tolerances and preferences and work with the pointers that you know will stick. If you make a positive health change and practice it regularly for at least 6 weeks it will become habit, shortly after you won't even have to think about your new healthy move because it will be your new "normal."
I challenge you to give it a try.

Final Thoughts

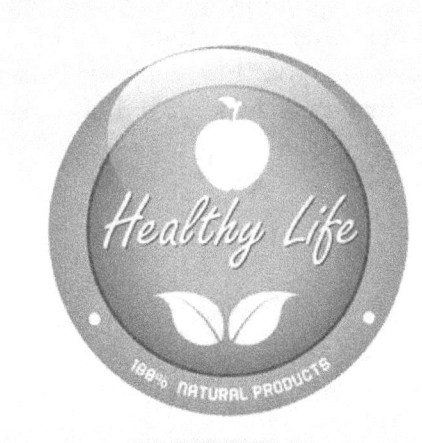

People end up packing on extra pounds for all sorts of controllable reasons. The key here is that for the most part weight gain is preventable and reversible. So if you really want to lose fat you can. But only you can decide that.

You can continue to make excuses or you can stop that crap and take action. I've shown you the reasons why we gain weight, given you the knowledge you need to understand fat, weight gain and how it fits into your life. I've also supplied you with the "know-how" to take action and get rid of your excess fat so that you can feel good about you, by increasing your energy levels, decreasing the risk for serious disease and increasing your self- confidence and overall belief in you.

Bottom line is it really doesn't matter how much I preach to you about fat loss or all the negatives associated with too much fat on your body. If you don't want to make the effort to change your thinking and make reasonable healthy lifestyle changes to help you lose fat and get healthy, then it's just not going to happen.

You are important as is your health and happiness. Set up a plan to start making better food choices and implement enjoyable regular exercise into your life regularly. This is only going to make your life that much better and I only see good in that! Are you ready to get started?

We have the choice to look for the positive or the negative in life. You can choose to lift someone up or to stomp on them. Writing is my passion and I work hard at it, with the goal of helping make people better. If you gain a new piece of knowledge, read something that makes you think, or perhaps even smile a few times, then I am happy and content!

Life's just too short not to tune into optimism. If your glass is half full, then I invite you to read my writing, and if you have a minute to spare when you're through, **I would appreciate your review.** This will help me better myself and my writing. I thank you in advance and appreciate you.

www.ingramcontent.com/pod-product-compliance
Lightning Source LLC
Chambersburg PA
CBHW070828290526
45795CB00002B/873